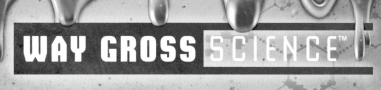

THE GROSS SCIENCE OF
ATHLETE'S FOOT

MARY-LANE KAMBERG

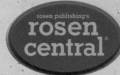

rosen publishing's
rosen
central

New York

For Chad Rohrback, a fun guy

Published in 2019 by The Rosen Publishing Group, Inc.
29 East 21st Street, New York, NY 10010

First Edition

Library of Congress Cataloging-in-Publication Data

Names: Kamberg, Mary-Lane, 1948– author.
Title: The gross science of athlete's foot / Mary-Lane Kamberg.
Description: New York : Rosen Central, 2019. | Series: Way gross science | Audience: Grades 5–8. | Includes bibliographical references and index.
Identifiers: LCCN 2017045963 | ISBN 9781508181590 (library bound) | ISBN 9781508181606 (paperback)
Subjects: LCSH: Athlete's foot—Juvenile literature. | Athlete's foot—Treatment—Juvenile literature.
Classification: LCC RL780 .K36 2019 | DDC 616.5/79—dc23
LC record available at https://lccn.loc.gov/2017045963

Manufactured in the United States of America

CONTENTS

INTRODUCTION

According to traditional Chinese medicine, the condition we now call athlete's foot was thought to be an illness of digestion. Athlete's foot is a contagious infection that most often appears as a rash between the toes. It can also cause scaly, flaky skin on the bottom of the foot or blisters anywhere on the foot.

Even though the rash, itching, and burning appeared on the feet, Chinese healers thought it was caused by stress and eating sugars and starches. They thought these factors made heat and moisture settle in the lower intestines. Treatment consisted of *shan zhi zi*, (gardenia fruit) and herbs to dry and cool the skin.

In the West, however, doctors once thought insect bites caused athlete's foot. Humans had suffered from the infection for centuries. But it was not described in medical terms until 1888. And not until 1908 did it appear in medical texts. The tiny organisms that actually cause athlete's foot were discovered two years later.

A common name for the condition (still often used today) is ringworm. Its name came from the circular pattern of the rash. No worm caused the infection, however. Instead, different fungi are at fault. Each causes different symptoms. Doctors group them under the name tinea. That name is followed by a term for where signs appear on the body. For example, tinea infection on the feet is called tinea pedis. On the arms, legs, or torso, it's tinea corporis. Tinea barbae occurs on the beard and face and tinea capitus on the head.

When scientists identified the cause of athlete's foot, they thought the condition rare. But its frequency increased during the 1900s. *Trichophyton rubrum*, one of the fungi that cause athlete's foot, first lived only in parts of Southeast Asia, Africa, and Australia. However, most

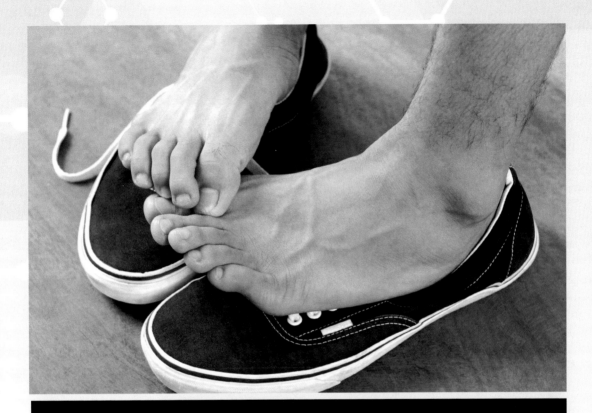

Athlete's foot sufferers deal with itchy, scaly, burning, or cracked skin, and sometimes blisters. Fortunately, treatments and cures are readily available.

people who lived in those areas avoided infection. They went barefoot. Their feet stayed cool and dry. The fungus had nowhere to grow.

However, as European nations sought to colonize these and other areas with warm, moist tropical climates, their shoe-wearing colonizers returned to their home countries carrying the fungus with them. It thrived in warm, damp shoes and socks. Some called the infection a "penalty of civilization."

It spread throughout Europe, especially when World War I brought mass movements of soldiers and refugees. Soldiers who wore socks and tightly laced, ankle-high boots for long periods caught it and brought it home with them. Refugees also spread the fungus to a wider area. The first reported case of tinea pedis in the United States occurred in Birmingham, Alabama, in the 1920s.

The presumed first use of the term "athlete's foot" appeared in a 1928 article in the *Literary Digest*. By the 1930s in America, the infection was thought a disease of the rich. They could afford leisure sports, which took place in swimming pools, country clubs, gymnasiums, and other places where athletes shared dressing rooms and showers.

Without a cure, doctors emphasized prevention. The first medically approved antifungal drug to hit the market was griseofulvin in the 1950s. It came as both a topical medicine applied on the skin and as an oral medication taken by mouth. Since then, more drugs have become available. However, athlete's foot remains a common—but usually curable—problem.

CHAPTER ONE

THE BIG ITCH

I t stings. It burns. Oozes. Crusts. Blisters. Maybe it swells. It can make the skin on the feet dry out, crack, flake, scale, or peel. Or turn red. Or raw. It can cause long, narrow splits in the skin between the toes. Or it can create a rash. Or cause thick, crumbly, or discolored toenails. Most of all, though, it itches!

It's athlete's foot. And, according to *Medical News Today*, you have a seven in ten chance of getting it sometime in your life. Amopé, a Canadian manufacturer of foot care products, estimates that at any time 15 to 25 percent of the world's population suffers from it.

Although it's most commonly seen in athletes, you don't have to play sports to catch it. Also called tinea pedis, or ringworm of the foot, athlete's foot is an infection caused not by a worm but by the most common types of foot fungi. Athlete's foot affects the upper layer of skin. And it thrives when the feet are warm, moist, or irritated.

TYPES OF ATHLETE'S FOOT

The three main types of athlete's foot affect different parts of the foot and cause different symptoms.

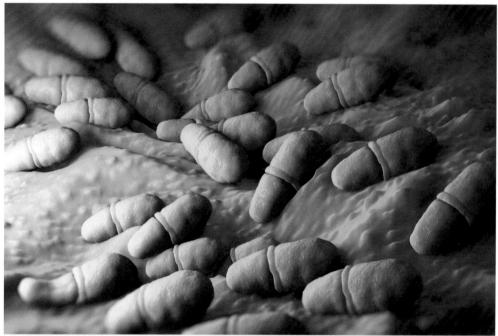

The fungi that cause athlete's foot lie dormant in the form of spores until warm, moist conditions "awaken" them. You can spread the spores without getting symptoms yourself.

Toe web infection affects the webbing, the skin between the toes. It often first affects the webbing between the fourth and fifth toes. In the beginning, the skin looks pale white and feels soft and moist. It itches, burns, and slightly smells. Then it turns scaly. It peels and cracks. If a bacterial infection sets in as well, the skin breaks down even more, and the odor turns foul. This type of infection is relatively easy to treat.

The vesicular infection is the least common form of athlete's foot. It starts with an outbreak of itchy, fluid-filled blisters under the skin. The blisters are gray with a dark peak surrounded by a red halo. Blisters usually first appear on the arch of the foot, but they can show up anywhere on the foot—even on the top. The same type of blisters can appear on the chest, arms, or fingers. Scratching the blisters easily bursts them.

That relieves the itch. However, bursting a blister spreads the infection. Bacterial infection may also accompany the fungus. The vesicular type of athlete's foot responds well to treatment.

Moccasin infection is the dry, scaly kind of athlete's foot. At first, dry skin with reddish edges and flakes covers the foot's surface—even

STINKY FEET

Not all foot conditions fall under the category of athlete's foot. One health problem often confused with it is pitted keratolysis. This bacterial infection affects the epidermis, the outer skin.

The skin on the heel and ball of the foot—and sometimes the palms or fingers—often looks like a honeycomb. Whitish skin is covered with clusters of punched-out pits. These pits may combine to create larger craters. In some cases, the skin on the sole has reddish areas. Pain or itching may be present.

The bacterium that causes it thrives in hot, humid weather. Pitted keratolysis is more common among men than women. It can happen at any age, but it's more common in older people. And it's often seen in athletes—hence the confusion with athlete's foot. It may also be a hazard of certain jobs. Farmers, sailors, fishermen, industrial workers, and military personnel are frequently infected. Workers in these careers may wear rubber boots or vinyl shoes that hold in moisture over long periods. Those who perform pedicures in spas and salons may also become infected.

Pitted keratolysis's most common symptoms are sweaty and very smelly feet. The foul odor comes from sulfur compounds produced by the bacterium. Treatment with topical antibiotics and antiseptics is usually successful.

extending to the entire foot in the shape of a moccasin shoe. The foot feels sore. Then the sole or heel becomes thick and cracks. Because this type of infection often has no other symptoms, those who have it may think they simply have dry skin. They may reach for moisturizers instead of antifungal medications. Moccasin athlete's foot is the hardest to treat and may last a long time.

IT'S COMPLICATED

Treating athlete's foot when symptoms first appear helps reduce the risk of complications. A complication is a new problem that results from an original infection. The first condition may become worse or show new symptoms. Complications of athlete's foot infection may be mild or more severe. Potentially mild complications include an allergic reaction to the fungus itself and the possibility of a repeat bout of infection after treatment.

Severe complications may involve an infection that spreads to the toenails. They crack, thicken, or crumble. Or fall off. Other, more severe complications include secondary bacterial infections caused by *Staphylococcus* or *Streptococcus* bacteria. These bacterial infections may include impetigo, ecthyma, and cellulitis. Such infections cause pain, swelling, fever, and pus drainage. Impetigo is a contagious skin infection. Ecthyma is a contagious form of impetigo that affects the area under the skin. Both impetigo and ecthyma cause blisters or sores on the face, neck, or hands.

Unlike impetigo and ecthyma, cellulitis is not contagious. Its main cause is the same bacteria as those infections, but other bacteria can also cause cellulitis. Cellulitis attacks both the skin and the tissues under the skin. Symptoms include pain, redness, swelling, tenderness, and burning in the affected area. Cellulitis often affects the legs, but it can happen anywhere on the body.

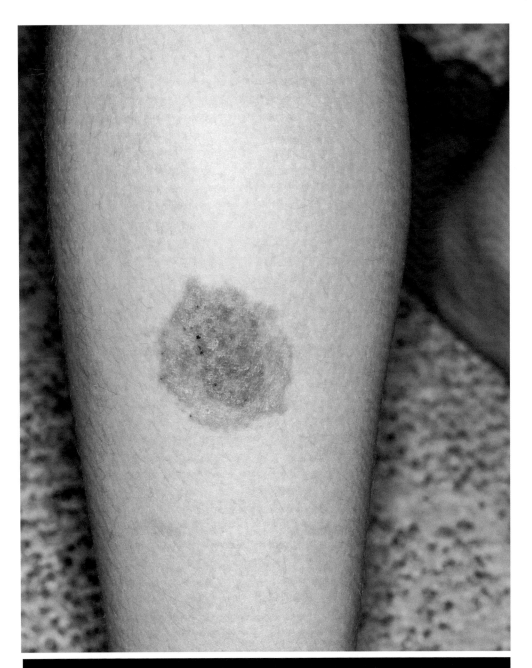

Impetigo is an infection caused by bacteria. The ring around the rash is sometimes confused with ringworm associated with athlete's foot.

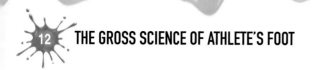

Another complication involves bacterial infections that spread to the lymph vessels or lymph nodes near the site of infection. The lymphatic system includes the tonsils, spleen, and thymus. The system protects the body from viruses and bacteria. Symptoms of lymphatic infection include chills, fever, and tender red streaks on the skin. This type of infection is easily treated. However, it can become serious without treatment.

Potentially severe complications of athlete's foot also include side effects from the very antifungal and antibacterial medications used to treat it.

MYTHS AND FACTS

Myth: Athlete's foot occurs only in athletes.

Fact: Athlete's foot is common among athletes—and named for them. But anyone can get it. Participating in sports often means feet spend a considerable time in warm, moist conditions such as sweaty socks and shoes during workouts and games. Also, the contagious fungi that cause athlete's foot easily spread on swimming pool decks, locker rooms, and shared shower floors.

Myth: Keeping feet clean by regular washing with soap and water prevents athlete's foot.

Fact: While it helps to keep feet clean, keeping them dry—especially between the toes—is more important. If an infection is present, soap and water won't kill the fungus that caused it. However, once treated, keeping feet clean and dry helps keep the infection from coming back.

Myth: You won't get athlete's foot if you don't walk around barefoot.

Fact: Walking barefoot on a surface that contains athlete's foot fungus is one way of becoming infected. However, the fungi also spread if you share towels, bed sheets, socks, shoes, or even nail clippers with an infected person. Walking barefoot and wearing sandals or open-toed shoes on uninfected surfaces actually helps prevent athlete's foot by keeping feet dry.

CHAPTER TWO

THE FUNGUS AMONG US

K nowing the cause of athlete's foot determines the proper treatment. Three different types of fungi may be responsible—alone or in combination. These include dermatophytes, yeasts, and molds. Some people are more prone to getting fungal infections than others. Unfortunately, medical experts don't yet know why.

Dermatophytes are the most common culprits involved in athlete's foot. They are moldlike parasites that grow on the skin, hair, and nails. The fungi feed on keratin, a protein found on the outer surfaces. Both toe-web and vesicular infections are caused by the *Trichophyton mentagrophyt* fungus. Moccasin infection is caused by *Trichophyton rubrum.*

Usually, the dryness of the outer layer of skin, along with the continual sloughing off of dead skin cells, keeps the fungi in check. However, trauma, irritation, or skin that has become soft by being exposed to long periods of moisture can provide the damp, warm conditions necessary for rapid reproduction. Colonies of the creatures form and spread. In addition to athlete's foot, dermatophytes cause nearly all fungal toenail infections.

RASH DECISIONS

Yeasts are fungi usually from the species *Candida*. They regularly reside on the skin and nails without causing trouble. However, illness, immune

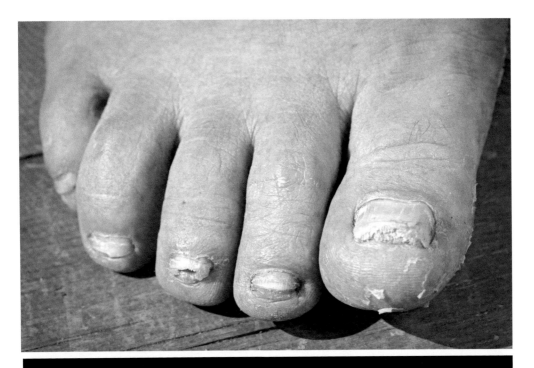

Treatment becomes difficult when toenails have fungal infections, which are almost always caused by dermatophyte fungi. Prescription medication may be necessary.

system problems, or antibiotic use can encourage too much yeast to grow and cause infection. Yeast can take advantage of athlete's foot and cause a secondary infection, particularly of the toenail beds and warm, moist areas of skin. The infections create splotches of a red, flat rash with rounded borders. Small, raised bumps filled with pus may also be present.

Molds are fungi that in rare cases cause infections that mimic athlete's foot. They are known as nondermatophytes. The most common molds that infect the feet are *Scopulariopsis brevicaulis* and *Scytalidinum dimidiatum*. These molds can also cause athlete's foot complications, especially of the toenails. While they can grow on the skin and nails, they're more commonly found in soil. They aren't contagious.

JOCK ITCH

Fungal infection of the groin, inner thighs, and buttocks areas is caused by the same fungi as athlete's foot. Its official medical name is tinea cruris, also known as ringworm or jock itch. This infection often spreads from infected feet. An infected person scratches their feet and at some point, touches their groin area.

Jock itch is most common in men and adolescent boys. However, men and women of any age can get it. The fungus loves such moist, damp environments as public showers, swimming pool decks, and locker rooms. Like athlete's foot, people who play sports aren't the only ones infected with it.

A good way to prevent jock itch if you have athlete's foot is to first dry the groin area after showering. Dry the feet last, being careful to completely dry between the toes. Wash the towel before reusing it. You should also put on socks before underwear to help prevent spores from jumping onto the fabric on its way past the feet. Along with towels, wash all socks, underwear, workout clothes, and athletic supporters after each use. Add chlorine bleach to the wash cycle when doing white loads of laundry.

STEPPING OUT

Fungi reproduce by creating spores that remain on the skin or travel through the air onto shoes, socks, bath mats, floors, and other surfaces. Spores are one-celled reproductive bodies similar to seeds. Spores can grow into mature fungi under warm, moist conditions. They have thick walls and save energy with a low metabolic rate. They can survive for more than a year under clean, dry conditions. Until warm, moist conditions exist, spores stay harmless. However, if a warm, moist environment

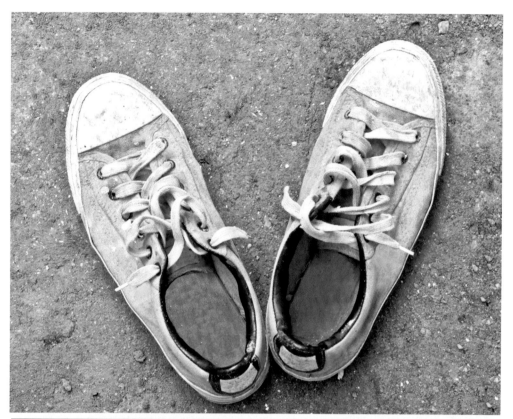

Fungal spores can "lie in wait" up to a year in a cool, dry place like old sneakers. If exposed to warmth and moisture, the spores "awaken" and cause infection.

presents itself, the spores become active, mature fungi that can cause infection.

The fungi that cause athlete's foot are highly contagious. They can spread from toe to toe, as well as to the soles and sides of the foot. They spread through touching the infected area of skin. For instance, scratching the rash helps it spread to other parts of the foot. The fungi can also move from one person to another in the same way. The infection also spreads through contact with clothes, socks, shoes, bed sheets, and towels used by an infected person.

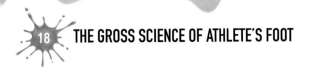
MY CAT HAS ATHLETE'S PAW

You can catch athlete's foot from your family pet and farm animals. The same fungi that infect humans also affect cats, dogs, and guinea pigs. Cows, goats, and horses can also get it. The infection usually is called ringworm in animals. The infection falls under the heading of a zoonotic disease. A zoonotic disease is one that can pass from animals to humans.

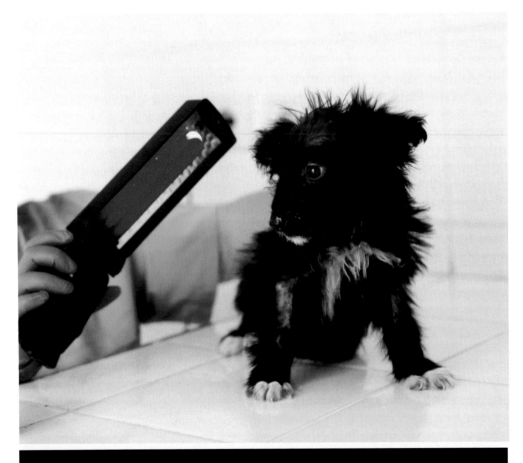

Dogs, cats, and other animals can contract the same infection that causes athlete's foot in humans. Veterinarians usually call the infection ringworm when it occurs in animals.

In animals, hair loss is a common sign of infection. The bald spots are flaky, crusty, circular areas with red central rings. In cats, they appear on the head, ears, and upper legs. The infection can also look like dandruff. The animal may react to the condition by continually gnawing its paws. The infection is highly contagious to other animals and humans. In fact, cats can carry the fungal spores without showing any symptoms. Infected dogs, however, almost always display the signs.

According to MedicineNet, as many as 13 percent of human tinea infections come from the same fungus that causes ringworm in cats. Also according to MedicineNet, in between 30 percent and 70 percent of households that have a pet cat with the infection, at least one human will also have symptoms.

Animals catch the ringworm fungi the same way humans do. They spread through direct contact with an infected animal or through bedding or other items the infected animal used. Kittens younger than one year and old cats are most likely to develop the condition. So are longhaired cats and those with suppressed immune systems, such as those with feline leukemia, also known as FeLV.

Veterinarians treat animals with ringworm using prescription shampoo or antifungal ointments. If you have other pets, ask the vet if they should also be bathed. Be sure to wash your hands with soap and water after bathing or touching the animal.

In severe cases, an oral medication is needed. Disinfecting the home is also important to keep the infection from spreading to others in the household or from coming back. Wash the pet's bedding and toys with antifungal disinfectant. If you can't disinfect such items as carpeted pet trees, throw them away. Because the fungal spores can survive in the hair and skin cells the animal sheds, be sure to vacuum often.

CHAPTER THREE

STEPS IN THE RIGHT DIRECTION

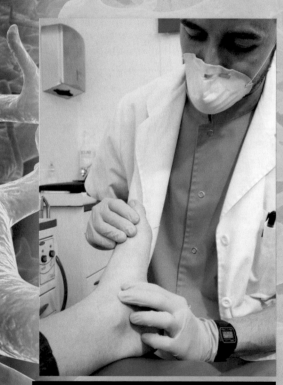

Sometimes, athlete's foot is so severe it requires prescriptions from podiatrists, who treat foot ailments.

Athlete's foot is usually easy to treat. In fact, if you notice it when it first appears, you can take care of it yourself at home. Caution: if you have diabetes and think you have athlete's foot, seek immediate treatment from a podiatrist or other doctor. Diabetes is a serious disease that involves lack of control of the amount of sugar in the blood and can affect the skin. A podiatrist is a health care professional who specializes in treating injuries and diseases and disorders of the feet.

If you don't have diabetes, start with an over-the-counter (OTC) antifungal medication when symptoms first appear. OTC medication is available at drug stores, grocery stores, and other retailers without a prescription. Start with topical medicine. Topical medicine is medicine that is applied to the skin at the site of the infection. Antifungal topical medicine comes in powder, liquid, spray, and cream forms. When choosing a product, know the medication's active ingredients. Look for the brands below, which contain specific antifungal ingredients:

- Exelderm (sulconazole)
- Kz Cream (ketoconazole)
- Lamisil AT (terbinafine)
- Lotrimin (clotrimazole)
- Lotrimin Ultra (butenafine)
- Micatin, Desenex (miconazole)
- Monistat, M-Zole, Micatin (miconazole)
- Spectrazole, Ecostatin (econazole)
- Tinactin (tolnaftate)

Look for anti-itch properties as well as antifungal ones. However, never use products that contain cortisone unless prescribed by a doctor.

WHAT TO LOOK FOR

When choosing an OTC product, consider the price. Look for an affordable choice. Some other factors to consider include the way the product is applied. Athlete's foot is painful. So look for applications that need only a gentle touch. Avoid products that sting when applied. Sometimes those with strong fragrance will cause the infected skin to sting.

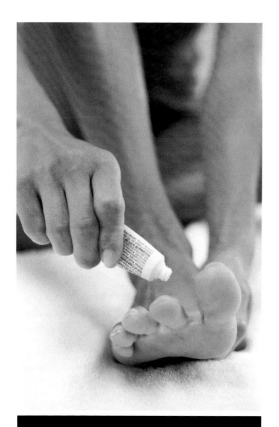

Over-the-counter antifungal cream may be all that's necessary to treat a new case of athlete's foot.

MAKE IT STOP!

Some easy home remedies can relieve the itching, burning, stinging, and blistering of athlete's foot while you wait for the antifungal medicine to finish its job. Relieving these symptoms helps keep you from scratching the infected skin and spreading the infection.

- Baking soda paste—Reduce itching, burning, and stinging with a baking soda and water paste. Place one tablespoon of baking soda on a saucer. Add water a little at a time until you have a thick paste. Spread the paste between the toes and onto other infected areas. Let the paste dry for five to ten minutes. Rinse with cool water. Dry thoroughly with a clean towel. Use two or three times a day.
- Apple cider vinegar and water—Dry up blisters and reduce itch by soaking the feet in a mixture of half apple cider vinegar and half water. Soak for ten minutes once a day.
- Saltwater soak—For blisters, mix two teaspoons of salt and one quart of warm water. Soak the feet for five to ten minutes several times a day.

Please note: These remedies relieve only the symptoms of athlete's foot. They may not kill the fungi that cause athlete's foot.

Instead, look for a product that soothes the burning and itching that the infection causes.

If the product contains a moisturizer, be sure the skin can readily absorb it. Otherwise, when cream sits on the skin, it provides a moist environment that encourages fungus growth. Also, consider how long the product takes to work. Some products clear up athlete's foot in a week or two. Others take as long as eight weeks. To reduce the risk of reinfection, keep using the product even after symptoms disappear. Always follow package instructions. For additional help choosing an OTC treatment, ask a pharmacist. If the infection won't go away, gets worse, or comes back, see a health-care professional.

NATURE WALKS

If you like, you can choose natural remedies to kill the fungus and clear up athlete's foot. Plain, unsweetened yogurt with a live culture can kill fungus and prevent its spread. Yogurt contains live acidophilus, a bacterium that helps maintain an acidic environment that kills yeast—one of the types of fungus that causes athlete's foot.

Yogurt is effective in two ways. You can eat one cup of yogurt two to four times a day to keep the fungus in check. And you can use a cotton swab to spread the yogurt directly onto the infected skin. Let it dry. Then rinse with warm water and towel dry. Continue eating yogurt and applying it to the feet until the infection completely disappears.

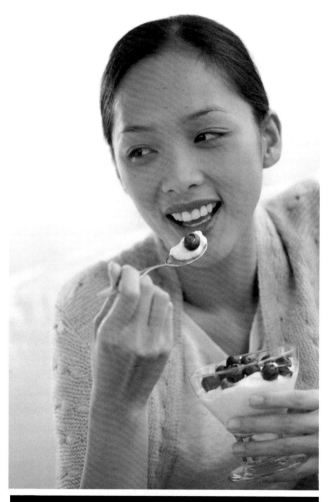

Plain, unsweetened yogurt with live acidophilus treats athlete's foot caused by yeast. Eat it or apply it to the skin to maintain an acidic environment yeast can't tolerate.

Mustard powder also contains acid that kills fungus. Fill a shallow pan with warm water. Add one teaspoon of mustard powder or a few drops of mustard oil to the pan. Soak your feet for thirty minutes twice daily until the skin is clear.

As every horror movie lover knows, garlic keeps away vampires. It can also treat athlete's foot. Garlic contains an antifungal compound called ajoene. Ajoene is a natural antifungal and antibacterial agent. Like yogurt, garlic is effective both as a food and as a topical treatment. However, you'll have to eat a lot of it. Add one or two cloves to food to help speed the healing process. Or make a paste by crushing one garlic clove and adding two or three drops of olive oil. Apply the paste to the skin and wait thirty minutes. Wash with warm water and antifungal soap. Dry with a clean towel. Use once per day for several weeks.

NATURAL OILS

Essential oils are oils that come from plants and have the plants' characteristic fragrances. They are used in the manufacture of perfumes, flavors, and pharmaceuticals. Three essential oils successfully treat athlete's foot. Tea tree oil, lavender oil, and coconut oil may be beneficial.

Tea tree oil comes from the *Melaleuca alternifolia* tree found in Australia. The oil contains natural antiseptic, antifungal, and antibacterial agents. It kills some athlete's foot infections. The *Australian Journal of Dermatology* reported effective treatment in 64 percent of participants with athlete's foot in a study using a 50 percent solution of the oil mixed with 50 percent of another substance. In another study in South Wales, Australia, researchers saw complete cures in 64 percent of subjects using a 50 percent solution. They also saw improved symptoms in 72 percent of participants who used only a 25 percent solution. Unfortunately, tea tree oil causes skin inflammation in some patients. To use it, mix a solution of half tea tree oil and half olive oil or 75 percent tea tree oil and 25 percent aloe vera gel. Rub it onto the infected area twice a day for six to eight weeks.

To get the best effects of tea tree oil add, a solution of ten drops of tea tree oil and ten drops of lavender oil to one cup of aloe vera juice, witch hazel, or a nongreasy, unscented lotion. Apply to the infected skin three times a day until the infection clears. You can also make a foot soak by adding ten drops of lavender oil and seven drops of tea tree oil to a container filled with hot water. The container should be large enough for both feet. Soak for twenty minutes.

Finally, coconut oil is a saturated fat that can help increase the body's immune function. The capric acid found in coconut oil kills the fungi that cause yeast infections, including those that cause athlete's foot. Coconut oil can be mixed with tea tree oil for foot-bath treatment of athlete's foot. Mix five or six drops of tea tree oil with one tablespoon of coconut oil and rub onto the feet. Use twice a day for four weeks.

Natural remedies can treat athlete's foot, but they need at least three weeks to work. If symptoms worsen or if you develop an allergic skin inflammation, stop using them and consult your health-care provider.

CHAPTER FOUR

THE DOCTOR IS IN

Some cases of athlete's foot go away in a short time. Others resist treatment. Your own efforts to heal your skin infection on the feet just may not work. Or they may take too long. Or you may not be treating it correctly. You may turn out to have something other than athlete's foot. It's time to call a doctor or other health-care provider.

You have many choices in the kind of provider to see. Dermatologists specialize in skin ailments. Podiatrists specialize in injuries and diseases of the feet. You can also see a pediatrician, who treats children, or a family practice doctor who sees patients of all ages. Adults can see internal medicine physicians, who treat adults for diseases that don't require surgery.

You can also choose a physician's assistant or nurse practitioner. A physician's assistant practices medicine as part of a team with physicians, surgeons, and other health-care workers. Some work in doctors' offices. They examine, diagnose, and treat patients. Nurse practitioners consult with physicians to determine the best way to treat a patient. They often work in pediatricians' offices, as well as with doctors in other specialties. Nurse practitioners have more education and training than licensed practical nurses and registered nurses. Nurse practitioners can prescribe drugs and order laboratory tests.

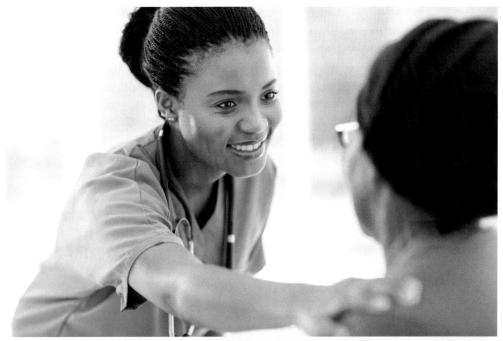

Health-care providers who can treat athlete's foot include several types of physicians, as well as nurse practitioners and physician's assistants.

CALL ME

Seek professional help when you have athlete's foot along with any of these conditions:

- You have diabetes or a disease that involves poor circulation. If so, you're at higher risk of developing a secondary bacterial infection of the foot or leg than those without those conditions.
- You have a weak immune system. You may need help fighting the infection.
- You have blisters on your feet, or pus oozes from them.

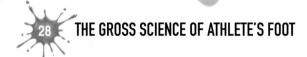
- The skin on your feet is severely cracking, scaling, or peeling.
- Symptoms seem to be spreading.
- You have increased pain, swelling, redness, tenderness, or burning.
- You see red streaks coming out of the infected area.
- You have a fever of 100.4 degrees Fahrenheit (38 degrees Celsius) or higher without the presence of another illness.
- Your athlete's foot symptoms don't improve after two weeks of use of an OTC antifungal treatment.
- The symptoms aren't completely cured after four weeks of using

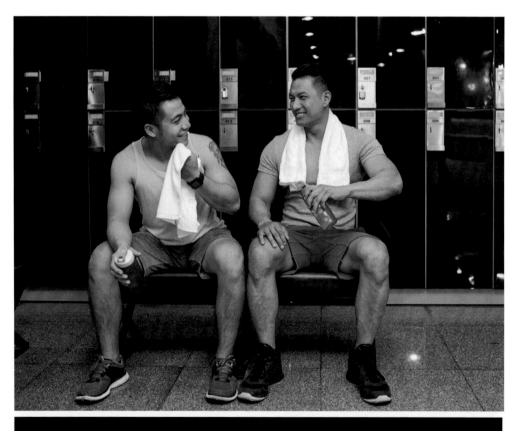

Locker rooms are places where fungi that cause athlete's foot are common. The fungi can spread from floors but also from shared towels and clothing.

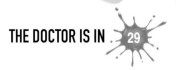

nonprescription drugs.
- Symptoms are severe or frequently return after treatment.

WHAT IS IT?

Health-care workers usually diagnose athlete's foot simply by looking at the skin and listening to the patient. You'll want to report when you first noticed symptoms and what the skin looked like at onset. Also tell the provider whether the rash itches, burns, or causes pain. If you've tried treatments on your own, the provider will want to know what you've done and whether symptoms improved, got worse, or stayed the same. He or she may also want to know whether any others in your family have the same signs. Be sure to let him or her know if you have been swimming or spending time in saunas, locker rooms, or other warm, moist places where fungi are likely to spread.

WHAT IT'S NOT

In addition to pitted keratolysis, some other conditions may be confused with athlete's foot. A mild infection not caused by athlete's foot fungi can present the same or similar symptoms. These include such diagnoses as dermatitis, psoriasis, and eczema.

Dermatitis makes skin red, swollen, and sore. It can also cause small blisters. The cause of dermatitis can be skin irritation from something in the environment. Or it can come from an allergic reaction. Psoriasis is a disease that creates patches of red, scaly skin with white scabs of dead skin. Like athlete's foot, psoriasis itches. However, unlike athlete's foot, it's not contagious. Eczema is not contagious either. Like athlete's foot, eczema causes severe itching and

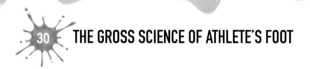

burning. It causes redness and small, oozing blisters to appear. The blisters can become scaly, crusty, or hard.

TESTING SKIN SAMPLES

Lab tests can help health-care providers identify whether a skin infection is athlete's foot. The most common is called the KOH test. KOH is the formula for the compound potassium hydroxide. In the periodic table, K stands for potassium, O stands for oxygen, and H stands for hydrogen. To perform a KOH test, a health-care provider collects a sample of the infected skin from the patient. A scalpel or the edge of a glass slide is used to gently scrape off some skin. A lab worker then places the sample in a

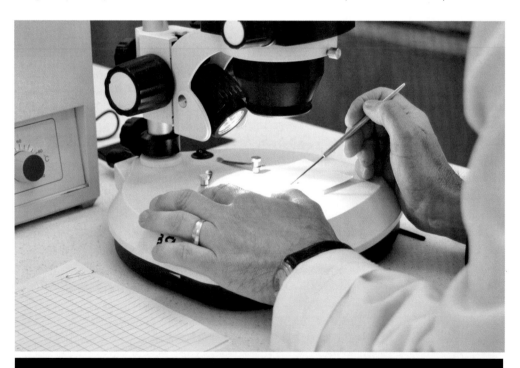

Sometimes, lab testing of skin samples is needed to identify the type of infection so the proper treatment can be prescribed.

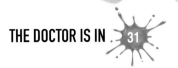

potassium hydroxide solution. The solution kills all the cells except for the fungus. The lab worker then looks at the fungus under a microscope to see what kind it is.

Another way to identify the cause of skin conditions is through a culture to see if a fungus is present. If so, the test shows which fungus it is. In the lab, a worker places a skin sample on a substance that promotes the growth of fungi. If a fungus grows on the substance, the lab worker looks at it through a microscope or performs chemical tests to see what kind of fungus grew.

A skin biopsy may be ordered in rare cases of athlete's foot. However, a biopsy is usually used to look for skin cancer. A biopsy is a test that removes cells or tissue to check for disease. Again, a small piece of infected skin is removed. It may be soaked in formaldehyde or simply placed in a sterile container. A lab worker then examines the sample under a microscope.

In addition to these tests to identify the cause of a skin infection, other tests may help health-care providers decide which medicine to use. For example, the doctor may order a test to see whether bacteria are resistant to a particular drug.

10 GREAT QUESTIONS TO ASK
A HEALTH-CARE PROFESSIONAL

1. What caused my symptoms?
2. What tests do I need to diagnose the problem?
3. How long will this condition last?
4. Will it go away by itself?
5. What treatment do you recommend?
6. Does the medicine have a generic version?
7. How should I take care of my skin while I'm using the medicine?
8. How can I keep the infection from spreading?
9. Once it clears up, can I get it again?
10. What preventive steps can I take to avoid another infection?

CHAPTER FIVE

BEST FOOT FORWARD

A fter athlete's foot goes away, it can return. There are some important steps to help keep that from happening. First, be sure to keep taking antifungal medicine for the prescribed time. Even if symptoms clear, some fungal spores may stay alive. They can flare up and reinfect the skin.

Second, keep feet dry, especially between the toes. If you had a toe web infection, dust the feet with powder and place lamb's wool between the toes. You can get lamb's wool at most pharmacies. Third, keep your clothes clean. Use the hottest water that's safe for the fabrics. When possible, add bleach to the wash cycle. Wear socks, swimsuits, T-shirts, and workout clothes only once between washings.

Fourth, replace flip-flops or shower shoes you wore while the infection was present. Finally, practice preventive measures so you'll resist

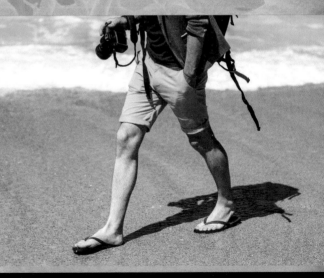

If you wore flip-flops or shower shoes while you had athlete's foot, throw them away! Those nasty spores might still cling to the shoes and cause reinfection.

athlete's foot if you are again exposed to the fungi. These include never walking barefoot in locker rooms or around pools, making sure to dry your feet completely after washing, and wearing breathable socks that dry quickly.

HAPPY FEET

Prevention is the best medicine. You can't always prevent athlete's foot, but you'll have a better chance with healthy foot care habits. The most

ARE YOU AT RISK?

Some people are at greater risk for developing athlete's foot than others. In fact, people can spread athlete's foot without showing signs of infection themselves. Experts don't know the reason. However, they have noticed factors for those at higher risk.

- Gender—Men are more likely than women to get athlete's foot.
- Location—Those who live in a warm, damp climate have a higher risk than those who live in cool, dry places.
- History—People with a history of athlete's foot or other fungal infections are more likely than others to get it again.
- General health—People with diabetes, cancer, or other illnesses that impair the immune system are more likely than others to become infected.
- Age—Older children and young adults get athlete's foot more often than young children.

important way is to keep feet, shoes, and socks clean, dry, and cool. Wearing shoes and socks combines natural body heat with the moisture of perspiration—the perfect habitat for fungal growth.

So walk barefoot as much as possible. According to *Medical News Today,* only about 0.75 percent of people who regularly go barefoot get athlete's foot. However, do wear flip-flops on pool decks, in locker rooms, and in public showers.

Wash your feet with soap and water twice a day in the hottest water possible. Completely dry them after— especially between the toes. Avoid sharing towels.

Use antifungal powder on the feet each day. Or use a homemade lavender foot spray. Place ten drops each of lavender oil and tea tree oil into one cup of distilled water. (You can substitute ten drops of myrrh oil

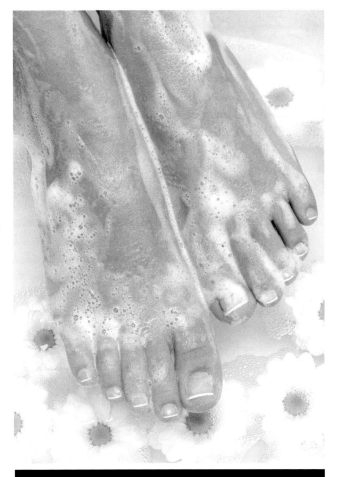

To prevent athlete's foot or reinfection after it clears up, wash feet with soap and water twice a day. Be sure to dry completely, especially between the toes.

for the tea tree oil.) Stir. Pour the solution into a clean spray bottle. Spray the feet and dry before putting on socks and shoes.

Finally, choose your socks and shoes wisely.

SHOE SHOPPING

Always wear light, well-ventilated shoes. Avoid thick ones. Go shoe shopping in the afternoon or evening. Your feet are slightly bigger during these times of day. You can be sure the shoes won't feel too tight later if you try them on when your feet are largest. A good rule of thumb is to be sure you can wiggle the toes when the shoe is on.

Avoid shoes made of plastic, vinyl, or rubber. Those materials hold in heat. Look instead for shoes made of such breathable materials as leather or canvas. Remove shoes as soon as possible after exercising or playing sports. Switch to sandals or flip-flops. Let sports shoes dry out for at least twenty-four hours before wearing again. The same goes for regular shoes. Never wear the same pair two days in a row. Give them the best chance of completely drying between uses.

With the prevention of athlete's foot in mind, shoe manufacturers have taken steps to maximize airflow in their sneakers. Up until the 1980s, they punched air holes—called ventilation eyelets—into the sides of their shoes. The eyelets have since been replaced by mesh side panels. Mesh fabric allows for more airflow than eyelets. And the more mesh, the better. While the frame of the shoe may be made of plastic or leather, the upper part of many sneakers today are made almost entirely of mesh. They provide maximum ventilation to discourage fungal growth.

SOCKS GALORE!

If you're trying to prevent athlete's foot, socks can be your worst enemy—or your first line of defense. Certainly, sweaty socks are nobody's friend. Change them when they get damp, especially after exercise. Wash them in hot water with bleach.

However, socks can help keep feet dry. Some experts advise wearing socks made of natural fibers like cotton or wool. Others recommend

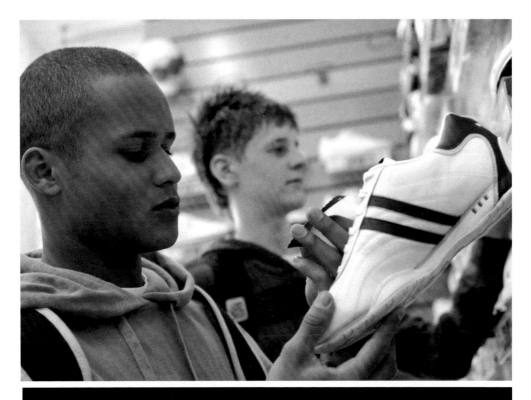

While everyone has a favorite pair of shoes they just can't part with, buying new shoes can help prevent the spread of athlete's foot.

socks made of synthetic fibers that wick away moisture. Wicking fabric is designed to pull away moisture from the skin. The moisture moves to the outside of the garment, where it evaporates. Without wicking, moisture from sweat and body heat are trapped between the skin and the clothing. Keeping moisture away from the skin reduces the risk of blisters and athlete's foot.

The following brands make wicking socks: Balega, Champion, Columbia, Dickies, Nike, Saucony, and Under Armour. They are made from blends of polyester, nylon, spandex, elastine, rubber, and cotton. Avoid ridged socks and those with tight, elastic tops. These features can irritate skin or reduce blood flow.

When choosing socks and shoes, look for the American Podiatric Medical Association (APMA) Seal of Acceptance. The seal recognizes socks, shoes, insoles, materials, and equipment that promote good foot health. A committee of podiatrists reviews each product. The item must allow for normal foot function, be useful, ensure safety, and have good quality control in its production. The seal is awarded for a three-year period and products can be reevaluated.

Following good preventive practices can help keep the fungus that causes athlete's foot in check. If, despite all efforts, an infection occurs, it's usually easy to treat. Over-the-counter medicine can cure most cases, especially if used soon after symptoms appear. Home remedies can control the itching and burning that comes with the infection. Severe cases and those with complications may require prescription medication under the supervision of a health-care provider. The good news is that most cases of athlete's foot are mild and disappear relatively quickly.

GLOSSARY

acidophilus A bacterium found in yogurt with a live culture that kills the fungi that cause athlete's foot.

ajoene A natural antifungal and antibacterial agent found in garlic.

biopsy A test that removes and examines cells or tissue to check for disease.

capric acid A fat found in coconut oil that kills the fungi that cause yeast infections, including those that cause athlete's foot.

dander Small flakes of skin that shed from the coats or feathers of animals (including humans).

dermatologist A doctor who specializes in diseases and infections of the skin.

dermatophyte A parasitic, moldlike fungus that grows on the skin, hair, or nails.

diabetes A serious disease that involves lack of control of the amount of sugar in the blood.

epidermis The outer layer of skin. The four tiers of the epidermis include the bottom level that creates new, living cells. As these cells move toward the outer body through two more levels, they flatten and dry out. When they reach the top level, they flake off.

moccasin-type athlete's foot A fungal infection caused by *Trichophyton rubrum* and marked by dry, flakey skin that affects the foot's surface, resulting in a rash that appears around the foot in a pattern that would be covered by a moccasin shoe.

nurse practitioner A nurse with more education and training than a licensed practical nurse and a registered nurse. Nurse practitioners can prescribe drugs and order laboratory tests.

oral medicine Medicine that is swallowed in pill or liquid form.

over-the-counter (OTC) medication A medication available without a prescription.

physician's assistant A health-care worker who practices on a team with physicians, surgeons, and other health-care workers. They are qualified to examine, diagnose, and treat patients.

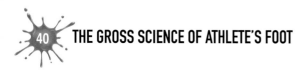

pitted keratolysis A bacterial infection of the outer skin often confused with athlete's foot.

podiatrist A health-care professional who specializes in treating injuries and diseases of the feet.

toe web athlete's foot A type of fungal infection caused by the *Trichophyton mentagrophyt* fungus that first affects the skin between the toes—usually between the fourth and fifth toes.

topical medicine Medicine applied directly to the skin at the site of infection.

ventilation eyelets Air holes punched into the sides of sneakers to aid in increasing airflow.

vesicular athlete's foot A type of fungal infection caused by the *Trichophyton mentagrophyt* fungus and marked by an outbreak of itchy, fluid-filled blisters under the skin. They usually first appear on the arch of the foot but can show up anywhere on the foot—even on the top.

zoonotic disease A disease, like athlete's foot, that can spread from animals to humans.

FOR MORE INFORMATION

American Academy of Dermatology (AAD)
PO Box 4014
Schaumburg, IL 60168
(888) 462-3376
Website: https://www.aad.org
Facebook: @AADmember
Twitter: @AADmember
Founded in 1938, the AAD represents more than nineteen thousand
    practicing dermatologists in the United States and internationally. It
    provides education, research, and advocacy to promote excellence in
    patient care.

American Academy of Podiatric Sports Medicine (AAPSM)
3121 NE 26th Street
(352) 620-8562
Website: http://www.aapsm.org
The AAPSM provides programs for research and education. It also seeks
    to increase the awareness of the profession of podiatric sports medi-
    cine and support students studying in the field.

American Podiatric Medical Association (APMA)
9312 Old Georgetown Road
Bethesda, MD 20814
(800) 366-8227
Website: http://www.apma.org
Facebook: @theAPMA
Twitter: @APMA
The APMA supports prevention and management of lower extremity
    sports-related injuries. It also provides public education to increase
    awareness of foot and ankle health.

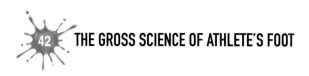

Canadian Federation of Podiatric Medicine (CFPM)
200 King Street S
Waterloo, ON N2J 1P9
Canada
(888) 706-4444
Website: http://www.podiatryinfocanada.ca/Public/Home.aspx
The CFPM is a national association of chiropodists and podiatrists in
    Canada. It represents its members with government agencies and
    professional organizations. It also offers educational opportunities and
    support for practitioners.

Canadian Podiatric Medical Association (CPMA)
120 Carlton Street
Suite 305
Toronto, ON M5A 4K2
Canada
(888)-220-3338
Website: http://www.podiatrycanada.org
The CPMA is a nonprofit association of more than four hundred
    Canadian foot specialists. It seeks to improve the podiatry specialty
    and to publicize the importance of foot health care among Canadians.

National Podiatric Medical Association
1706 E. 87th Street
Chicago, IL 60617
(773) 374-5300
Website: http://www.npmaonline.org
The National Podiatric Medical Association is dedicated to attracting and
    supporting minorities and disadvantaged individuals in the field of
    podiatry. It provides financial support, as well as placement in resi-
    dency, clinical, and teaching roles.

FOR FURTHER READING

Aldersmith, Herbert. *Ringworm: Its Diagnosis and Treatment.* Charleston, SC: Nabu Press, 2012.

Banks, Scott J. *Natural Cures for Dummies.* Hoboken, NJ: John Wiley & Sons, 2015.

Bowman, Katy. *Simple Steps to Foot Pain Relief: The New Science of Healthy Feet.* Dallas, TX: BenBella Press, 2016.

Chiodo, Christopher P., and James P. Ioli. *Healthy Feet: Preventing and Treating Common Foot Problems.* Cambridge, MA: Harvard Health Publications, 2015.

Elston, Ruth. *How to Use Tea Tree Oil—90 Great Ways to Use Nature's "Medicine Cabinet in a Bottle."* San Diego, CA: Better Life Books, 2013.

Fullem, Brian. *The Runner's Guide to Healthy Feet and Ankles: Simple Steps to Prevent Injury and Run Stronger.* New York, NY: Skyhorse Publishing, 2015.

Sanchez, Anita. *Itch! Everything You Didn't Want to Know About What Makes You Scratch.* Boston, MA: HMH Books for Young Readers, 2018.

Smith, William J. *On Ringworm: An Inquiry Into the Pathology, Causes and Treatment.* South Yarra, Victoria, Australia: Leopold Classic Library, 2015.

Turner, John P. *Ringworm and Its Successful Treatment.* South Yarra, Victoria, Australia: Leopold Classic Library, 2016.

Vonhof, John. *Fixing Your Feet: Injury Prevention and Treatments for Athletes.* Birmingham, AL: Wilderness Press, 2016.

BIBLIOGRAPHY

Amopé. "Playing the Field: A Sportsperson's Guide to Athlete's Foot." Retrieved July 29, 2017. http://www.amope.ca/en/all-about-feet /on-the-move/playing-the-field-a-sportsperson-s-guide-to-athlete-s -foot.

Aronson, Anna. "What Is Nystatin Cream?" *Livestrong.com*, August 16, 2013. http://www.livestrong.com /article/145491-what-is-nystatin-cream.

Boston Children's Hospital. "Athlete's Foot (Tinea Pedis)." *Young Men's Health.com*, July 13, 2017. http://youngmenshealthsite.org/guides /athletes-foot/.

Burgess, Patrice, and E. Gregory Thompson. "Athlete's Foot." *WebMD*, September 25, 2014. http://www.webmd.com /skin-problems-and-treatments/tc/athletes-foot-topic-overview#1.

Doheny, Kathleen. "Ringworm or Candida: What's the Difference?" *WebMD*, April 06, 2012. http://www.webmd.com /skin-problems-and-treatments/features/ringworm-or-candida#1.

Jordaan, H. F. and Sean J. Pincus. "Athlete's Foot." *Health 24*, February 13, 2013. http://www.health24.com/Medical/Fee t/Common-foot-problems/Athletes-foot-20120721.

Lee, Kevin. "Guide to Using Tea Tree Oil and Athlete's Foot." *Healthy Oil Planet*, Retrieved July 29, 2017. https://www.healthy-oil-planet.com /tea-tree-oil-and-athletes-foot.html.

Legacy Pediatrics. "Athlete's Foot (Tinea Pedis)." Retrieved July 29, 2017. https://www.legacypediatrics.com/parent-guide/skin-care /athletes-foot/.

Leigh, Katie. "Home Remedies to Cure Foot Fungus." *Livestrong.com*, August 16, 2013. http://www.livestrong.com /article/117656-home-remedies-cure-foot-fungus.

Lowe, Caitlynn. "Fissures & Athlete's Feet Treatment." *Livestrong.com*, July 18, 2017. http://www.livestrong.com /article/556573-fissures-athletes-feet-treatment.

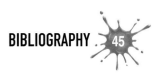

Mayo Clinic staff. "Athlete's Foot." *Mayo Clinic*, August 19, 2016. http://www.mayoclinic.org/diseases-conditions/athletes-foot/home/ovc-20235864.

Nordqvis, Christian. "Athlete's foot: Symptoms, causes, and treatments." *Medical News Today*, February 27, 2017. http://www.medicalnewstoday.com/articles/261244.php.

Oakley, Amanda. "Pitted Keratolysis." *Derm Net New Zealand*, April 2016. https://www.dermnetnz.org/topics/pitted-keratolysis.

Roizman, Tracey, D. C. "Coconut Oil for Athlete's Foot." *Livestrong.com*, January 7, 2016. http://www.livestrong.com/article/533213-coconut-oil-for-athletes-foot.

Stöppler, Melissa Conrad. "Catching Ringworm from Pets." *MedicineNet.com*, December 1, 2014. http://www.medicinenet.com/script/main/art.asp?articlekey=82553.

Sullivan, Debra. "Athlete's Foot." *Healthline.com*, October 19, 2015. http://www.healthline.com/health/athletes-foot#Treatment6?utm_source=ask&utm_medium=referral&utm_campaign=asksearch.

Supplement Police. "Athletes Foot Fungus Treatment Guide." Retrieved July 29, 2017. https://supplementpolice.com/health-guides/athletes-foot.

Tang, Kay. "Sneakers That Have Good Ventilation for Athlete's Food." *Livestrong.com*, December 28, 2015. http://www.livestrong.com/article/406886-sneakers-that-have-good-ventilation-for-athletes-feet.

INDEX

A

acidophilus, 23
American Podiatric Medical Association (APMA) Seal of Acceptance, 38
Amopé, 7
antibiotic, 15

B

biopsy, 31

C

Candida, 14
causes, of athlete's foot, 7–13
cellulitis, 10
Chinese medicine, 4
complications, of athlete's foot, 10, 12, 15, 38
cortisone, 21
culture, 23, 31

D

dermatitis, 29
dermatologists, 26
dermatophytes, 14
diabetes, 20, 27, 34

E

ecthyma, 10
eczema, 29
essential oils, 24–25, 35
Europe, 5

F

foot care, 34-35

G

garlic, 24
griseofulvin, 6

H

health-care professionals, 26–32
home remedies, 22, 38

I

impetigo, 10–11
insect bite, 4

J

jock itch, 16

K

keratin, 14
KOH test, 30

L

lymphatic system, 12

M

moccasin infection, 9, 14
mold, 14, 15
mustard powder, 24

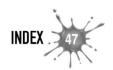

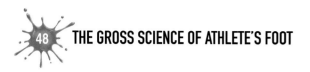

ABOUT THE AUTHOR

Mary-Lane Kamberg has written extensively on health topics for *Current Health, Healthy Kids, Kansas City Magazine,* and *Your Health and Safety.* She is the author of the following additional books on health topics for Rosen Publishing: *When a Parent Has PTSD, Chlamydia, Self-Esteem and Body Image, Teen Pregnancy and Motherhood,* and *Sports Concussions* (In the News). She is coleader of the Kansas City Writers Group and lives in Olathe, Kansas.

PHOTO CREDITS

Cover Miroslav Lukic/Shutterstock.com, pp. 7, 14, 20, 26, 33 (background) Stocktrek Images/Getty Images; pp. 1, 4–5 (background) matthew25/Shutterstock.com; p. 5 Pedalist/Shutterstock.com; p. 8 Royaltystockphoto.com/Shutterstock.com; p. 11 Education Images/ Universal Images Group/Getty Images; p. 15 Elena11/Shutterstock.com; p. 17 Cbenjasuwan/Shutterstock.com; p. 18 Ershova_Veronika/iStock /Thinkstock; p. 20 BEELDPHOTO/Shutterstock.com; p. 21 PhotoAlto /Odilon Dimier/Getty Images; p. 23 tmcphotos/Shutterstock.com; p. 27 Michael Jung/Shutterstock.com; p. 28 DragonImages/iStock/Thinkstock; p. 30 Tony4urban/Shutterstock.com; p. 33 Ross Helen/Shutterstock .com; p. 35 Valua Vitaly/Shutterstock.com; p. 37 Peter Cade/Iconica /Getty Images.

Design: Michael Moy; Editor: Bethany Bryan; Photo Research: Sherri Jackson